ANEMIA

EXPLORING THE ENDLESS POSSIBILITIES OF
ANEMIA TREATMENTS

DR. J. SIMON

Table of Contents

INTRODUCTION

A decrease in the quantity of hemoglobin in the blood or a deficiency of red blood cells is known as anemia, a frequent medical ailment. Hemoglobin is a necessary protein found in red blood cells that binds to oxygen and carries it to various human tissues and organs. Low hemoglobin or red blood cell levels impair the body's ability to carry oxygen, which can result in a range of symptoms.

There are several types of anemia, and each has its own characteristics and causes. The most common kinds include iron deficiency anemia, vitamin deficiency anemia, and anemia linked to chronic diseases.

Although anemia can produce many symptoms, weakness, tiredness, pale complexion, lightheadedness, and difficulty concentrating are the most prevalent ones. Numerous underlying conditions, including inadequate food, chronic diseases, genetics, and some medical procedures, can result in anemia.

Blood tests are frequently used in diagnosis to determine hemoglobin levels, red blood cell count, and other pertinent characteristics. The path of treatment for anemia will depend on its specific kind and cause, but it typically involves treating the underlying causes with dietary changes, iron supplements, or other medical treatments.

Anemia can affect people of different ages and backgrounds, and its consequences on overall health can range from minor to severe. Early detection and efficient treatment are necessary to reduce symptoms and prevent complications.

CHAPTER ONE

Understanding anemia requires an understanding of the intricate relationships that exist between oxygen, hemoglobin, and red blood cells in the body. Let's examine more closely:

The purpose of red blood cells (RBCs) is:

Red blood cells, or erythrocytes, are responsible for carrying oxygen from the lungs to the rest of the body and carbon dioxide from the lungs back to the lungs for expiration.

The Value of Red Blood Cells

A molecule called hemoglobin is found in red blood cells; when blood flows, it binds to oxygen in the lungs and delivers it to tissues and organs. Iron is required for hemoglobin to bind oxygen.

Types of Anemia:

Iron-deficiency anemia is the most common type. It is mostly caused by insufficient iron intake or absorption, which lowers the generation of hemoglobin.

Vitamin B12 and folic acid deficiencies, which are necessary for the production of red blood cells, can result in vitamin deficiency anemia.

Chronic disease-related anemia: This condition affects the body's ability to use iron for the production of hemoglobin and is linked to conditions including inflammation and recurrent infections.

Causes and Risk Factors:

Deficits in nutrition: Insufficient consumption of folic acid, iron, or vitamin B12.

Chronic Illnesses: Conditions include inflammatory diseases and chronic renal disease might affect the generation of red blood cells.

Genetic Factors: Two instances of hereditary anemias include sickle cell anemia and thalassemia.

Warning signs:

Fatigue: Due to a decrease in the blood's capacity to carry oxygen.

Pale skin can result from low hemoglobin and red blood cell counts.

Breathlessness: The body's inability to get the oxygen it requires.

Weakness and vertigo: Linked to insufficient oxygenation of the brain and muscles.

One of the most crucial blood tests for the diagnosis of anemia is a complete blood count (CBC). These tests evaluate hemoglobin levels, red blood cell count, and other pertinent factors.

Counseling:

Iron or vitamin supplements: Depending on the type of anemia, supplements may be recommended to address nutritional deficiencies.

Dietary Adjustments: Increasing the intake of foods high in iron, folic acid, and vitamin B12.

Treating underlying causes can include controlling chronic conditions or addressing inherited factors that lead to anemia.

Knowing the different causes, symptoms, and treatment options for anemia is essential to understanding the condition. It emphasizes the significance of keeping a balanced and nutrient-dense diet, treating underlying medical issues, and, in some situations, taking supplements in order to support healthy red blood cell generation and hemoglobin function. Regular medical exams and monitoring are crucial for the proper management and prevention of anemia-related issues.

Anemia comes in a variety of forms, each with its own causes and characteristics. Here are some examples of common anemias:

Iron deficiency anemia:

Cause: Persistent blood loss (from menstruation, gastrointestinal bleeding, etc.) or inadequate ingestion of iron or absorption from food.

Features: Low iron levels prevent the body from producing hemoglobin and red blood cells. It is the type of anemia that is most prevalent worldwide.

Anemia Vitamin Deficiency:

Deficiency in Vitamin B12 Causing Anemia:

Cause: Inadequate intake of vitamin B12 or problems absorbing it, often associated with gastrointestinal difficulties or diseases such as pernicious anemia.

Features: Vitamin B12 is necessary for the synthesis of red blood cells. Deficiencies may lead to big, immature red blood cells.

A lack of folic acid resulting in anemia:

Cause: Inadequate ingestion or poor absorption of folic acid (vitamin B9).

Features: Folic acid is necessary for the synthesis of DNA during the creation of red blood cells. One possible cause of abnormally big red blood cells is a deficit.

Anemia from Chronic Disease:

Cause: Rheumatoid arthritis, inflammatory bowel disease, infectious illnesses, and chronic renal disease are a few examples of underlying chronic disorders.

Features: The body's inability to use iron for hemoglobin formation is caused by inflammation, which leads to anemia.

Hemolytic anemia:

Cause: Genetic problems, autoimmune diseases, or certain drugs can cause hemolysis, or the accelerated breakdown of red blood cells.

Characteristics: Reduced red blood cell viability and increased demand for production of red blood cells.

A sickle cell anemia:

Cause: A genetic mutation that causes hemoglobin S, an abnormal form of hemoglobin, to be produced.

Characteristics: Red blood cells become sickle-shaped and harden, which can lead to discomfort, organ damage, and an increased risk of infection.

Thalassemia:

Cause: An inherited genetic disorder that prevents the production of hemoglobin.

Features: Anemia is caused by a decreased synthesis of healthy hemoglobin. There are two primary forms of thalassemia, beta and alpha, which differ in severity.

Aplastic Anemia:

Cause: Damage to the bone marrow, often caused by autoimmune illnesses, radiation, chemotherapy, and certain medications.

Features: Decreased platelet, white blood, and red blood cell production.

Anemia Hemorrhagic:

Cause: Blood loss, either acute or chronic, as a result of trauma, surgery, or gastrointestinal bleeding.

Features: A reduction in the overall volume of red blood cells in circulation causes anemia.

Determining the best course of action for treatment and management requires an understanding of the particular kind of anemia. In order to promote the generation of red blood cells, it frequently entails treating the underlying reason, offering dietary support, and, in certain situations, using medication.

CHAPTER TWO

Typical Reasons

Understanding the causes of anemia is essential for an efficient diagnosis and course of treatment. Following are a few typical causes of anemia:

Iron Insufficiency:

Insufficient Dietary Intake: A diet deficient in foods high in iron.

Poor Iron Absorption: Illnesses of the intestines, such as celiac disease, can make it difficult for the body to absorb iron.

Blood Loss: Prolonged bleeding, frequently from stomach hemorrhage, ulcers, or menstruation in women.

Inadequate intake of vitamins:

Deficiency in vitamin B12 can be caused by inadequate food consumption, gastrointestinal issues, or pernicious anemia, an inflammatory disease that affects B12 absorption.

Folic Acid Deficiency: Inadequate folic acid consumption, typically associated with diets deficient in particular fruits and green leafy vegetables.

Chronic Illnesses:

Inflammatory Disorders: Chronic disease-related anemia can be brought on by illnesses such as rheumatoid arthritis, inflammatory bowel disease, or chronic kidney disease.

Chronic Infections: Prolonged infections can impede the synthesis of red blood cells.

Conditions Inherited and Genetic:

An inherited genetic condition called sickle cell anemia causes aberrant hemoglobin levels.

Thalassemia: Genetic conditions that impair hemoglobin synthesis.

Red blood cell destruction, or hemolysis:

Conditions that are inherited include G6PD deficiency and hereditary spherocytosis.

In autoimmune hemolytic anemia, red blood cells are unintentionally attacked and destroyed by the immune system.

Aplastic Anemia:

Radiation, chemotherapy, some medicines, and autoimmune illnesses can all damage bone marrow.

Anemia Hemorrhagic:

Trauma, surgery, gastrointestinal bleeding, or illnesses such as hemorrhoids can cause either acute or chronic bleeding.

Chronic Kidney Disease:

Reduced Erythropoietin synthesis: Erythropoietin is a hormone that promotes the synthesis of red blood cells, and it is produced in part by the kidneys. Anemia can be brought on by renal impairment.

Being pregnant:

Increased Blood Volume: The body requires more iron and other nutrients during pregnancy, which raises the possibility of iron-deficiency anemia.

Syndromes of Malabsorption:

Celiac disease: Iron and B vitamins may be poorly absorbed as a result of gluten intolerance.

Substances:

A number of pharmaceuticals, including nonsteroidal anti-inflammatory drugs (NSAIDs), have been linked to anemia and gastrointestinal bleeding.

Determining the precise cause of anemia is essential to creating a customized treatment strategy. It frequently entails treating underlying illnesses, dietary inadequacies, or genetic predispositions that result in either decreased red blood cell production or greater red blood cell destruction. To identify the underlying cause of anemia, a comprehensive medical examination and diagnostic procedures are necessary.

Signs and symptoms

Numerous symptoms can accompany anemia, and the degree and arrangement of these symptoms might change based on the underlying cause and general health of the patient. The following are typical signs of anemia:

Weakness and Fatigue:

feeling abnormally weak or exhausted, even after getting enough sleep.

Light Skin:

Skin tone, particularly apparent on the cheeks, mouth, and nail beds.

Breathiness Shortness:

breathlessness or difficulty breathing, especially when exercising.

Fast Heartbeat:

palpitations or an elevated heart rate as a result of the heart trying to make up for the blood's decreased ability to deliver oxygen.

Feeling lightheaded or dizzy:

feeling lightheaded or vertigo, especially after rising up fast.

Cold Feet and Hands:

feeling of coolness in the limbs as a result of reduced oxygen and blood flow.

Headache:

frequent or ongoing headaches, frequently linked to a decreased oxygen supply in the brain.

Cognitive Problems:

mental haze, forgetfulness, or trouble focusing.

Intolerance:

heightened irritation or mood swings.

Hair Loss:

Hair thinning or loss, possibly due to decreased blood supply to the hair follicles.

Nails growing ridges or becoming brittle and weak.

Intolerance to cold:

Feeling extremely cold, even in warm weather.

Sensation for Inert Substances (Pica):

unusual desires for materials such as starch, ice, or clay, which could be a sign of an iron shortage.

Inflamed or Sore Tongue:

tongue inflammation, discomfort, or swelling (known as glossitis).

It's crucial to remember that anemia symptoms might be hard to notice at first because they can be mild and appear gradually. Sometimes people may not exhibit any symptoms at all until their anemia gets worse. It is imperative that you get medical attention for a correct diagnosis and suitable treatment if you suspect you have anemia or if you are experiencing any of these symptoms.

Identification

An extensive process is used to diagnose anemia, including a physical examination, a medical history, and specialized blood testing. An outline of the anemia diagnostic procedure is provided below:

Health Background:

Symptom Assessment: The medical professional will ask about any indicators of anemia, including weakness, exhaustion, and shortness of breath.

Personal and Family History: It is important to know about drug regimens, dietary practices, medical problems, and any family history of anemia or similar diseases.

Physical Assessment:

Observation: The medical professional might notice physical symptoms like pallor, a fast heartbeat, or bleeding indications.

Examining the heart and lungs to look for signs of respiratory distress and an increased heart rate.

Examining the abdomen for discomfort or enlargement of any organs.

Blood Tests:

Complete Blood Count (CBC): This examination counts the platelets, white blood cells, and red blood cells in the blood. It offers details on the hemoglobin concentration and size of red blood cells.

Hemoglobin and Hematocrit Levels: The quantity of hemoglobin and the volume of red blood cells in the blood are indicated by these assays.

A peripheral blood smear is a microscopic analysis of a blood sample to determine the red blood cell's size, shape, and color. It aids in the identification of anomalies like sickle cell disease or peculiar cell morphologies.

Reticulocyte Count: This test determines the proportion of immature, young red blood cells and gives insight into the bone marrow's capacity to generate new red blood cells.

Iron Studies: These examinations measure ferritin, total iron-binding capacity (TIBC), and serum iron levels.

Levels of vitamin B12 and folate should be measured to look for vitamin deficiencies, particularly in cases with macrocytic anemia.

A peripheral blood smear is a microscopic analysis of a blood sample to determine the red blood cell's size, shape, and color. It aids in the identification of anomalies like sickle cell disease or peculiar cell morphologies.

Extra Examinations:

Bone Marrow Aspiration and Biopsy: Under some circumstances, a sample of bone marrow may be obtained to evaluate the bone marrow's capacity to produce blood cells.

Specialized Tests: Additional tests like autoimmune markers, hemoglobin electrophoresis, or genetic testing may be carried out based on the hypothesized cause of anemia.

The outcomes of these tests aid in identifying the kind and origin of anemia, assisting the medical professional in creating a customized treatment strategy. For an accurate diagnosis and efficient treatment, anyone exhibiting signs of anemia should have a complete examination performed by a medical specialist.

CHAPTER THREE

Strategies for Treatment

The goal of treating anemia is to increase hemoglobin and red blood cell synthesis while addressing the underlying cause. The kind and etiology of anemia determine the appropriate course of treatment. These are typical methods of treatment:

Supplementing with Iron:

Iron-Deficiency Anemia: Iron supplements may be recommended if low iron levels are the cause of the anemia. It's important to take them as prescribed and to talk to a healthcare professional about any possible adverse effects.

Supplements with vitamins:

Supplements containing vitamin B12 or folate may be advised for anemia brought on by these vitamin deficits. Injections may be required in specific circumstances.

Modifications to Diet:

Iron-Rich Foods: Promoting an iron-rich diet that includes foods like leafy green vegetables, lean meats, beans, and nuts.

Foods Rich in Vitamins: These include foods high in folate (leafy greens, legumes, fortified cereals) and vitamin B12 (mcat, fish, dairy).

Handling of Concomitant Disorders:

treating and controlling any underlying illnesses, such as inflammatory diseases or chronic illnesses, that may be causing anemia.

Agents that Stimulate Erythropoiesis (ESAs):

In certain circumstances, ESAs may be administered to promote red blood cell formation, particularly in chronic kidney disease.

Transfusion of Blood:

A blood transfusion could be required in an emergency or for severe anemia in order to rapidly restore red blood cell counts.

Bone Marrow Inducing Agents:

Medication that encourages the bone marrow to create more blood cells may be taken into consideration in specific circumstances.

Modifications in Lifestyle:

Working with a licensed dietitian to ensure a diet rich in nutrients and well-balanced is known as nutritional counseling.

Taking care of contributing factors: Taking care of things like severe menstrual bleeding, gastrointestinal bleeding, or other blood loss sources.

Frequent Observation:

Blood testing and routine follow-up visits to track therapy response and make necessary intervention adjustments.

To find the best course of action for their particular kind of anemia, people with anemia must collaborate closely with their healthcare providers. Self-diagnosis and self-medication can be dangerous because proper diagnosis is necessary for efficient therapy. In order to enhance general health and quality of life, treatment success frequently entails a combination of medical interventions, lifestyle modifications, and treating the underlying causes.

Nutritional deficiencies are a major cause of anemia, and dietary treatments are essential in treating this condition. The following food plans can help with anemia:

Iron-Dense Foods:

Eat a range of foods high in iron in your diet. Among them are:

Lean meats include chicken, lamb, hog, and beef.

Fish: Particularly shellfish such as sardines, oysters, and clams.

Plant-Based Sources: Fortified cereals, tofu, and legumes (lentils, beans).

Nuts and Seeds: Almonds, sunflower, and pumpkin seeds.

Rich in Vitamin C Foods:

The iron that is contained in plant-based meals is called non-heme iron, and vitamin C helps to improve its absorption. Incorporate vitamin C-rich foods into your meals, such as:

Fruits with citrus skins (grapefruits, oranges, lemons).

fruit, such as blueberries, raspberries, and strawberries.

Mango, pineapple, melons, and kiwis.

Green Leafy Vegetables:

Add leafy, dark greens to your meals because they are high in iron and folate. Collard greens, Swiss chard, spinach, and kale are a few examples.

Foods fortified:

Select meals that are enriched with iron, such as pasta, bread, and cereals. Verify the labels to make sure additional iron is present.

Cut Proteins:

Choose sources of lean protein that are high in iron and other necessary nutrients:

fowl without a skin.

Fish.

lean beef or pork portions.

Eggs:

Heme iron, which is more readily absorbed by the body, is found in eggs. If you're not a vegan or vegetarian, include eggs in your diet.

Pulses and Legumes:

Rich in iron, beans, lentils, and chickpeas can be eaten as a side dish or added to soups, stews, and salads.

Whole Grains:

Go for whole grains because they have higher iron and other minerals. Quinoa, brown rice, and whole wheat are a few examples.

Fruits that are dried:

Dried fruits that are high in iron, such as prunes, raisins, and apricots, can make healthy snacks.

Steer Clear of Iron Inhibitors:

A few foods may prevent the absorption of iron. Steer clear of them when eating meals high in iron. Tea, coffee, and foods high in calcium are a few examples.

Never forget how important it is to have a balanced diet and make sure you're getting a range of nutrients. To build a customized dietary plan that takes into account your individual needs and dietary preferences, it is advisable to speak with a healthcare provider or a certified dietitian if you have been diagnosed with anemia or if you have suspicions about it. When paired with medical measures, dietary changes can play a major role in controlling and reversing nutritionally associated anemia.

Avoidance

A healthy lifestyle, dietary decisions that promote sufficient nutrient intake, and management of potential risk factors are all important in preventing anemia. Here are a few precautions to take:

A well-rounded diet

Eat a diet high in iron, vitamin B12, and folate that is well-balanced. Eat a range of foods from various food groups, including fish, poultry, dairy, fruits, vegetables, whole grains, legumes, and lean meats.

Enhancement of Iron Absorption:

Eat foods high in vitamin C along with foods high in iron to improve the absorption of non-heme iron. For instance, incorporate vitamin C-rich veggies, berries, and citrus fruits into your meals.

Steer clear of iron inhibitors:

Be aware of drugs that may prevent the absorption of iron. Steer clear of tea and coffee right before or after iron-rich meals, and take calcium supplements sparingly.

Foods fortified with iron:

Include items like bread, pasta, and cereal that have been fortified with iron in your diet. Make sure the product labels indicate that iron has been added.

Supplementing with vitamins:

If you are susceptible to vitamin deficits (e.g., folate or B12), see a healthcare provider before taking any supplements.

Frequent Medical Examinations:

Keep an eye on your general health and look for any potential risk factors or early indicators of anemia by scheduling routine check-ups.

Handle Long-Term Illnesses:

Collaborate closely with your healthcare team to properly manage any chronic diseases you may have, such as inflammatory disorders or chronic renal disease, which may contribute to anemia.

Screening While Expectant:

Due to their elevated risk, pregnant women should have regular anemia screenings. Iron and folic acid-containing prenatal vitamins are frequently advised.

Preventing Abnormal Blood Loss:

Take precautions to avoid excessive blood loss, such as using safe sexual practices to avoid STDs and getting medical help right away if you experience any unusual bleeding.

Mild Exercise:

Regularly partake in mild physical activity, as it enhances general health and wellness. Be sure to speak with your doctor before beginning a new fitness program.

Give Up Smoking:

If you smoke, think about giving it up. Anemia can be exacerbated by smoking's effects on red blood cell formation.

Limit Consumption of Alcohol:

Drinking too much alcohol can affect how well some minerals, including iron, are absorbed. Moderation is the key.

It's crucial to remember that different prevention tactics may be used based on a person's age, health state, and unique risk factors. It is best to speak with a healthcare provider if you have questions regarding anemia or its risk factors so they can provide you with individualized advice and suggestions based on your particular health profile.

CONCLUSION

In summary, anemia is a frequent disorder marked by a lack of red blood cells or a reduction in hemoglobin levels, which lowers the blood's ability to carry oxygen. Numerous variables, such as genetics, chronic illnesses, malnutrition, and other medical disorders, might contribute to this syndrome.

Anemia can cause a variety of symptoms, such as weakness, exhaustion, pale complexion, and shortness of breath. An extensive medical evaluation, comprising a complete medical history, physical examination, and specialized blood tests, is necessary to diagnose anemia.

In order to treat the underlying cause, treatment methods may involve managing contributory factors, supplementing, and changing one's diet. A well-balanced diet, iron-rich foods, and vitamin supplements are essential for the management of anemia, particularly when it is associated with nutritional deficits.

A healthy lifestyle, a balanced diet, staying away from iron inhibitors, controlling chronic illnesses, and getting medical help when needed are all examples of preventive strategies. Early detection and prevention of anemia are facilitated by routine health examinations and knowledge of relevant risk factors.

All things considered, knowledge of anemia, its causes, and practical management techniques enables people to actively maintain ideal blood health. Anemia can be effectively managed or prevented by people with the right medical assistance, lifestyle modifications, and nutrition focus, all of which will enhance overall health and vigor.

THE END

9 798876 237132